Water Bath Canning and Preserving Guide for Beginners

The Basics of Water Bath Canning

By

Eanraig Harris

Table of Contents

CHAPTER 1

Introduction

1.1. Why Water Bath Canning?

Water bath canning is a time-honored method of food preservation that has been employed by generations of home cooks and food enthusiasts. It is a process that involves sealing jars of food with hot water to create a vacuum seal, effectively preserving the contents for extended periods. While it may seem like a traditional technique in today's fast-paced world, water bath canning offers several compelling reasons for its continued popularity and relevance.

Preservation of Seasonal Abundance: One of the primary reasons for embracing water bath canning is its ability to capture the flavors and nutrition of seasonal produce at their peak. Whether it's the sweetness of ripe summer peaches or the tang of freshly harvested tomatoes, canning allows you to enjoy these flavors year-round. By preserving surplus fruits and vegetables, you can reduce waste and make the most of your garden or local farmers' market.

Homemade Goodness: Water bath canning empowers you to take control of the ingredients that go into your preserved foods. You can adjust the sugar, salt, and spices to suit your taste and dietary preferences. This level of customization ensures that your canned goods are not only delicious but also free from artificial additives and preservatives, making them healthier and safer options for you and your family.

Cost-Effective: Canning is a cost-effective way to build a pantry stocked with nutritious and tasty foods. By purchasing produce when it's in season and abundant, you can save money compared to buying commercially canned items year-round. Canning also reduces the need for frequent grocery trips, which is particularly valuable when certain ingredients are not always readily available.

Gifts from the Heart: Home-canned goods make for thoughtful and personalized gifts. Whether it's a jar of homemade jam, a batch of pickles, or a collection of sauces and salsas, these handcrafted items carry a sense of care and love that store-bought gifts often lack. Sharing your canned creations with friends and family becomes a gesture of warmth and consideration.

1.2. Benefits of Preserving Food

Food preservation, as practiced through methods like water bath canning, extends well beyond the convenience of year-round availability. It offers a multitude of benefits that go far beyond the kitchen:

Long-Term Storage: Preserved foods have a significantly longer shelf life than fresh produce. This is crucial for ensuring food security and being prepared for emergencies. Having a well-stocked pantry can be a lifesaver during times of food scarcity or natural disasters.

Reduced Food Waste: The issue of food waste is a global concern. By preserving surplus or excess food, you play a part in reducing this waste. It's a small but impactful step towards a more sustainable and environmentally responsible food system.

Nutritional Retention: Contrary to popular belief, the canning process can preserve the nutritional content of food. Properly canned fruits and vegetables maintain many of their vitamins, minerals, and antioxidants, making them a nutritious addition to your diet.

Economic Savings: Preserving your own food can lead to significant savings over time. It helps cut down on grocery bills, especially during times of high food prices or inflation. Additionally, it enables you to take advantage of sales and discounts on seasonal produce.

Customized Flavors: Canning allows you to experiment with flavors and create unique culinary combinations. You can craft your own recipes, fine-tune the taste, and enjoy one-of-a-kind creations that cater to your specific preferences.

1.3. Safety Precautions

Safety is paramount when it comes to canning and preserving food. While it's a rewarding and enjoyable hobby, it's essential to understand and adhere to safety precautions to ensure that your canned goods are free from contamination and safe for consumption.

Proper Equipment: Using the right canning equipment is crucial. This includes canning jars, lids, bands, and a water bath canner. Ensure that your equipment is in good condition, with no cracks or chips, to prevent any potential issues with sealing and preserving your food.

Sanitation: Maintain a high level of cleanliness throughout the canning process. Thoroughly wash and sterilize your canning jars, lids, and utensils to prevent the introduction of harmful microorganisms. Pay attention to your workspace as well, keeping it clean and free of potential contaminants.

Follow Tested Recipes: Always use reliable, tested canning recipes from trusted sources. These recipes have been developed to provide the correct balance of acidity, sugar, and other components necessary for safe preservation. Deviating from tested recipes can result in unsafe food products.

Acidification: When canning low-acid foods like vegetables, it's crucial to add acid, typically in the form of vinegar or lemon juice, to ensure safe preservation. This acidification process inhibits the growth of harmful bacteria like botulism.

Processing Times and Temperatures: Pay close attention to the recommended processing times and temperatures for the specific foods you are canning. These guidelines are designed to destroy harmful microorganisms and pathogens, making the food safe for long-term storage.

Altitude Adjustments: If you live at a high altitude, you must make adjustments to your canning process to account for lower boiling points. This ensures that the food is processed at the correct temperature for safe preservation.

Testing Seals: After processing, carefully inspect the lids of your canned jars. A sealed lid should not flex or make a popping sound when pressed in the center. Any unsealed jars should not be stored and should be refrigerated and consumed promptly.

Record-Keeping: Keep records of your canning activities, including the date, recipe, and batch information. This can be invaluable in case you need to track the source of any issues with your preserved food.

Regular Inspections: Periodically inspect your canned goods for signs of spoilage, such as off-putting odors, mold growth, or unusual discoloration. If any of these issues are detected, discard the contents and do not consume.

By understanding the significance of safety precautions and following best practices, you can confidently engage in water bath canning, knowing that the food you preserve will be both delicious and safe for consumption. The journey of preserving your own food can be a rewarding and sustainable practice, and it begins with a firm commitment to safety and quality in your home canning endeavors.

CHAPTER 2

Getting Started

2.1. Equipment and Supplies

Before you embark on your water bath canning journey, it's essential to gather the right equipment and supplies to ensure a successful and safe canning experience. Proper tools and materials are key to achieving the best results. Here's what you need:

- **Water Bath Canner:** A large, deep pot with a lid and a rack that fits inside. This will be used to process the jars.

- **Canning Jars:** Glass jars with a two-part lid system consisting of a flat metal lid and a screw band.

Common sizes include pint, quart, and half-pint jars.

- **Canning Tools:** Invest in a set of canning tools that typically includes a jar lifter, magnetic lid lifter, bubble remover/headspace tool, and a wide-mouth funnel. These tools make the canning process safer and more convenient.

- **Thermometer:** A kitchen thermometer is useful for monitoring the temperature of your canning liquids.

- **Kitchen Timer:** Use a timer to keep track of processing times accurately.

- **Canning Recipes:** Start with tested and trusted canning recipes from reliable sources. These recipes are essential for ensuring food safety and flavor.

- **Fresh Ingredients:** Quality produce is at the heart of successful canning. Use the freshest fruits and vegetables, ideally picked at the peak of ripeness.

- **Vinegar and Lemon Juice:** When canning low-acid foods, you'll need acidification agents like white vinegar or lemon juice to maintain safe pH levels.

- **Salt and Sugar:** Depending on your recipes, you may need salt or sugar. Use canning and pickling salt, which is free from additives, and granulated sugar without anti-caking agents for best results.

- **Clean Towels and Cloths:** Keep plenty of clean towels or cloths on hand for wiping jar

rims, cleaning spills, and
handling hot jars.

- **Labels and Markers:** Label your canned goods with the contents and date of canning. This makes it easy to identify your preserved items later.

- **Storage Area:** Ensure you have a cool, dark, and dry place to store your canned goods after they've been processed.

Having the right equipment and supplies at your disposal will set you up for a smooth canning experience and make the process more efficient.

2.2. Choosing the Right Jars

Selecting the appropriate jars for water bath canning is a critical step in ensuring the success and safety of your preserved foods. Here's what you should consider when choosing jars:

- **Jar Size:** Choose the jar size that suits the type of food you're preserving and your intended use. Common sizes include pint (16 ounces), quart (32 ounces), and half-pint (8 ounces) jars. Smaller jars are great for jams and jellies, while larger ones are ideal for pickles and fruits.

- **Mouth Size:** Jars come in regular and wide-mouth options. Wide-mouth jars are more convenient for packing and retrieving items, especially larger or chunky foods.

- **Type of Glass:** Use only canning jars made of tempered glass designed for canning. These jars can withstand the temperature changes involved in canning. Avoid using recycled or re-purposed jars as they may not seal properly.

- **Two-Part Lid System:** Look for jars that come with a two-part lid system consisting of a flat metal lid and a screw band. The flat lid is necessary for sealing, and the screw band secures it in place. Check that both components are free from defects.

- **Check for Chips and Cracks:** Before use, inspect your jars for any chips, cracks, or defects in the glass, as these can prevent a proper seal.

- **Reusable or Disposable Lids:** Some canning lids are designed for one-time use, while others can be reused. Check the manufacturer's recommendations for the specific lids you choose.

- **Proper Sealing:** Ensure that the sealing area of your jars is clean and free from defects, as this is crucial for achieving a proper seal.

- **Preheat Jars:** To prevent thermal shock, preheat your jars by placing them in hot (not boiling) water before filling them with hot food. This helps to avoid jar breakage during processing.

- **Store Jars Properly:** Store your empty jars in a clean, dry place to prevent dust or contaminants from settling inside before use.

Choosing the right jars and properly preparing them is fundamental to the canning process. It ensures that your preserved foods remain safe and flavorful for an extended period.

2.3. Selecting Fresh Ingredients

The quality of your canned goods largely depends on the freshness and quality of the ingredients you use. When selecting fresh ingredients for canning, consider the following:

- **Peak Ripeness:** Whenever possible, use ingredients that are at their peak of ripeness. Fruits and vegetables harvested when they are fully ripe tend to be the most flavorful and nutritious. Check local produce markets, your own garden, or pick-your-own farms for the best options.

- **Quality Control:** Inspect the produce carefully, avoiding items with blemishes, bruises, or signs of decay. Use only the highest-quality ingredients to ensure that your canned goods are of the best possible quality.

- **Washing and Cleaning:** Before canning, wash and clean your fruits and vegetables thoroughly. Remove any dirt, insects, or debris. For some produce, peeling or blanching may be necessary before canning.

- **Trimming and Cutting:** Properly trim and cut your ingredients according to your chosen recipe. Some recipes require specific preparation, such as peeling, pitting, or slicing, so be sure to follow the instructions closely.

- **Consistency:** To achieve consistent canning results, try to maintain uniformity in the size and shape of your ingredients.

This ensures that all items in a batch are processed evenly.

- **Avoid Overripeness:** While ripe produce is ideal, avoid using ingredients that are overly ripe or starting to spoil. These may not can well and can negatively affect the quality of your canned goods.

- **Acidity:** When canning low-acid foods like vegetables, it's important to add acidification agents like white vinegar or lemon juice to maintain safe pH levels. Follow your canning recipe's guidelines for acidification.

Selecting fresh, high-quality ingredients is the foundation of creating delicious and safe canned goods. Whether you're canning fruits, vegetables, or other items, starting with

the best ingredients will ensure that
your preserved foods are a joy to
consume.

CHAPTER 3

The Basics of Water Bath Canning

3.1. Understanding the Canning Process

Before you start water bath canning, it's crucial to have a good understanding of the canning process. Here's what you need to know:

- **Heat Processing:** Water bath canning relies on heat processing to create a vacuum seal in canning jars. This seal prevents the growth of spoilage microorganisms and makes your preserved foods safe for long-term storage.

- **High-Acid vs. Low-Acid Foods:** It's important to differentiate between high-acid and low-acid foods when canning. High-acid foods, like most fruits and tomatoes, can be safely water bath canned because their natural acidity helps prevent bacterial growth. Low-acid foods, such as vegetables and meats, require acidification to ensure safe canning.

- **pH Levels:** For low-acid foods, pH levels play a significant role in safety. The goal is to maintain a pH level below 4.6. Acidification with lemon juice or vinegar helps achieve this.

- **Boiling Water Bath:** The water bath canner is essentially a large pot with a rack that holds canning jars. During processing, the jars are submerged in boiling water for a specific period to destroy microorganisms and enzymes that can cause spoilage.

- **Sealing Process:** After processing, as the jars cool, a vacuum seal forms. This seal pulls the lid down and creates an airtight environment inside the jar, preventing contamination and spoilage.

- **Headspace:** Leave the recommended amount of headspace (empty space at the top of the jar) as indicated in your recipe. Headspace ensures a proper seal and allows for food expansion during processing.

3.2. Preparing the Canning Area

Creating a clean and organized canning area is essential for an efficient and safe canning process. Here's what you should do to prepare your canning area:

- **Cleanliness:** Thoroughly clean your workspace, including countertops, cutting boards, utensils, and canning equipment. A clean environment reduces the risk of contamination.

- **Sanitization:** Properly sanitize your canning jars, lids, and utensils. You can do this by boiling the jars or running them through a dishwasher with a sanitize cycle. The lids can be simmered in hot (not boiling) water.

- **Water Bath Canner:** Fill the water bath canner with enough water to cover the jars with at least 1-2 inches of water. Heat the water, but do not bring it to a boil until you are ready to start processing.

- **Organization:** Gather all your equipment and ingredients within easy reach. This includes canning tools, labels, markers, and a kitchen timer.

- **Hot Jars:** Preheat your canning jars to prevent thermal shock. This can be done by placing the jars in hot (not boiling) water. Keep them hot until they're ready to be filled.

- **Keep a Towel Handy:** Have clean towels or cloths available to wipe the jar rims, clean up spills, and handle hot jars safely.

3.3. Preparing the Jars and Lids

Properly preparing the canning jars and lids is crucial for achieving a successful seal. Follow these steps for jar and lid preparation:

- **Inspect the Jars:** Before using the jars, inspect them for any cracks, chips, or defects. Damaged jars should not be used for canning, as they may not seal properly.

- **Wash the Jars:** Wash the jars, lids, and bands in hot, soapy water and rinse thoroughly. Ensure that there is no soap residue left on the jars.

- **Warm the Lids:** Place the flat metal lids in a pan of hot (not boiling) water to soften the sealing compound. Do not boil the lids, as excessive heat can compromise the seal.

- **Dry and Set Aside:** After washing, dry the jars and lids thoroughly with a clean, dry towel. Set them aside until you're ready to fill the jars.

- **Fill Jars Carefully:** When filling the jars with your prepared food, leave the recommended headspace as per your recipe. Be cautious not to overfill, as this can lead to sealing issues.

- **Wipe Jar Rims:** After filling each jar, wipe the rims clean with a clean, damp cloth to remove any food particles or residue. A clean rim is essential for a proper seal.

- **Apply Lids and Bands:** Place a pre-warmed lid on each jar, followed by a screw band. Screw the band on until it's fingertip tight – that is, snug but not overly tightened. Overtightening can prevent air from escaping during processing.

- **Set Jars in Canner:** Carefully place the filled and sealed jars in the rack of the preheated water bath canner. Make sure there's enough water to cover the jars by 1-2 inches.

Proper preparation and handling of jars and lids are vital for a successful canning process. Following these steps ensures that your canned goods will have a strong seal and remain safe for long-term storage.

CHAPTER 4

Water Bath Canning Step-by-Step

4.1. Preparing the Recipe

Before you start filling your jars, it's essential to have your canning recipe ready and follow it carefully. Here are the steps for preparing the recipe:

1. **Gather Ingredients:** Collect all the ingredients required for your canning recipe. These may include fresh produce, spices, vinegar, sugar, and any other components specified in your chosen recipe.

2. **Measure Ingredients:** Measure all ingredients precisely according to the recipe's

instructions. Accuracy in measuring is crucial for achieving the desired taste and safety.

3. **Cook the Recipe:** Follow your canning recipe's specific cooking instructions. This may involve simmering, boiling, or cooking the ingredients to the right consistency. Pay close attention to cooking times and temperatures to ensure the recipe is properly prepared.

4. **Stir and Skim:** While cooking, stir the recipe frequently to prevent sticking or burning. If necessary, skim off any foam or impurities that rise to the surface.

5. **Taste for Flavor:** Taste the recipe during cooking to ensure

it meets your flavor preferences. Adjust the seasonings if needed.

6. **Maintain Heat:** Keep the recipe hot. It's important to fill the jars with hot contents, as this promotes a successful seal and minimizes the risk of contamination.

4.2. Filling the Jars

Once your canning recipe is ready, it's time to fill the jars with the hot contents. Follow these steps for filling the jars:

1. **Remove a Jar:** Use a jar lifter to remove one preheated jar from the water bath canner. Empty the hot water from the jar back into the canner.

2. **Fill the Jar:** Using a wide-mouth funnel, carefully ladle or

pour the hot recipe into the jar.
Leave the recommended
headspace as specified in your
canning recipe. Typically, this is
around 1/4 to 1/2 inch, but it
may vary.

3. **Debubble the Jar:** Insert a
   bubble remover or headspace
   tool into the jar to release any
   trapped air bubbles. This helps
   ensure even distribution of
   contents and proper headspace.

4. **Wipe the Rim:** After
   debubbling, use a clean, damp
   cloth to wipe the rim of the jar to
   remove any food residue or
   liquid. A clean rim is essential
   for creating a secure seal.

5. **Apply Lid and Band:** Place a
   pre-warmed flat metal lid on the
   jar, and then screw a band onto
   the jar until it's fingertip tight.

The fingertip tightness allows air to escape during processing and prevents overtightening, which could interfere with the sealing process.

6. **Return to Canner:** Carefully place the filled and sealed jar back into the rack of the water bath canner. Ensure that the jar is positioned upright and doesn't touch the sides or bottom of the canner.

7. **Repeat the Process:** Continue filling jars, applying lids and bands, and placing them in the canner until all jars are filled or the canner is full.

4.3. Applying Lids and Bands

The final step in the water bath canning process is to apply lids and bands to your filled jars. Follow these steps for properly sealing your jars:

1. **Lid Application:** After filling and sealing each jar, apply a flat metal lid that has been pre-warmed in hot (not boiling) water. Place it on the jar's rim.

2. **Band Application:** Immediately screw on a band, also known as a screw band, until it's fingertip tight. Be cautious not to overtighten, as this can prevent the proper seal from forming.

3. **Check for Air Bubbles:** Check for any air bubbles by lightly tapping the side of the jar with a utensil or your fingertip. This

helps release any remaining air, ensuring the contents are evenly distributed.

4. **Repeat for All Jars:** Continue applying lids and bands to all the filled jars, one at a time, until you've sealed each one.

5. **Water Bath Canning:** After all the jars are filled, sealed, and placed in the water bath canner, ensure that there is enough water in the canner to cover the jars by 1-2 inches.

6. **Process Jars:** Place the lid on the canner and bring the water to a boil. Once boiling, start the timer for the specified processing time, as indicated in your canning recipe.

7. **Processing Time:** Maintain a gentle, rolling boil throughout the entire processing time, as

required by your recipe. The processing time may vary depending on the type of food and jar size.

8. **Cooling Jars:** After processing, turn off the heat and allow the jars to sit in the hot water for a few minutes. This helps prevent sudden temperature changes that can cause jar breakage.

9. **Remove Jars:** Using a jar lifter, carefully remove the jars from the canner and place them on a clean, dry towel or cooling rack. Leave space between the jars to allow for air circulation.

10. **Cooling and Sealing:** As the jars cool, you'll hear the satisfying "ping" of the lids sealing. This indicates a successful seal. Let the jars sit undisturbed for 12 to 24 hours to

cool and complete the sealing process.

11. **Check Seals:** After cooling, check each jar's seal by pressing the center of the lid. It should not flex or make a popping sound. Any unsealed jars should be refrigerated and consumed promptly.

Properly filling the jars, applying lids and bands, and following the processing steps are crucial for achieving safe and successful water bath canning results. Be patient during the cooling and sealing process, and make sure to store your sealed jars in a cool, dark, and dry place for long-term preservation.

4.4. Processing in the Water Bath Canner

Processing your jars in the water bath canner is a critical step to ensure the safety and preservation of your canned goods. Follow these steps to process your jars effectively:

1. **Boiling Water Bath:** Ensure the water bath canner is filled with enough hot water to cover the jars by at least 1-2 inches. The water should already be hot, but not necessarily boiling, when you place the jars inside.

2. **Rack Placement:** Carefully place the filled and sealed jars into the rack of the water bath canner. Make sure the jars are upright and evenly spaced, with enough room between them to allow water to circulate.

3. **Water Level Check:** Double-check that the water level is sufficient to cover the jars. Add more hot water if needed.

4. **Cover and Start the Timer:** Place the lid on the canner and turn up the heat to bring the water to a rolling boil. Once the water is boiling, start the timer for the specified processing time indicated in your canning recipe.

5. **Maintain a Boil:** It's important to maintain a consistent, gentle, rolling boil throughout the entire processing time. This ensures that the contents of the jars are thoroughly heated, destroying microorganisms and enzymes that can cause spoilage.

6. **Monitor the Timer:** Keep a close eye on the timer and make sure to process the jars for the

exact duration specified in your recipe. Processing times vary depending on the type of food and jar size.

7. **Adjust for Altitude:** If you live at a high altitude, it's important to adjust your processing time to account for the lower boiling point of water at higher elevations. Follow altitude adjustments provided in trusted canning resources.

4.5. Cooling and Sealing

After the processing time in the water bath canner, the final steps involve cooling and sealing your canned goods. Follow these steps to complete the water bath canning process:

1. **Turn Off the Heat:** After the jars have been processed for the

required time, turn off the heat under the water bath canner.

2. **Let Sit for a Few Minutes:** Allow the jars to sit in the hot water for a few minutes. This helps to prevent sudden temperature changes that could lead to jar breakage.

3. **Carefully Remove Jars:** Using a jar lifter, carefully lift the processed jars from the water bath canner. Place them on a clean, dry towel or cooling rack. Leave some space between the jars to allow for proper air circulation.

4. **Avoid Disturbing the Lids:** As the jars cool, you may hear a satisfying "ping" sound as the lids seal. This indicates a successful seal. Avoid moving or

pressing on the lids during this period.

5. **Cooling Time:** Allow the jars to cool undisturbed for 12 to 24 hours. During this time, the vacuum seal is formed as the contents contract and create an airtight seal.

6. **Check the Seals:** After the cooling period, check the seals on each jar by gently pressing the center of the lid. It should not flex or make a popping sound. Properly sealed jars will have a concave lid that doesn't move when pressed.

7. **Label and Store:** Once you have verified the seals, label each jar with its contents and the date of canning. Store your canned goods in a cool, dark,

and dry place for long-term preservation.

8. **Use Unsealed Jars Promptly:** If any jars didn't seal properly, store them in the refrigerator and use their contents promptly. They are not suitable for long-term storage.

Following these steps for processing in the water bath canner and ensuring a proper cooling and sealing process, you can confidently enjoy your home-canned goods, knowing they are safe and ready for long-term storage.

CHAPTER 5

Safety and Troubleshooting

5.1. Ensuring Proper Seal

A proper seal is crucial in water bath canning to ensure the safety and longevity of your preserved foods. Here's how to ensure a proper seal:

1. **Visual Inspection:** After the cooling period, visually inspect the lids on your canned jars. A properly sealed jar will have a concave, slightly depressed lid that doesn't flex when pressed in the center.

2. **Airtight Seal:** Check for airtightness by gently tapping the center of the lid with your

fingertip. A properly sealed lid should not make a popping or clicking sound when pressed. If it's sealed well, it will stay firm and not move.

3. **Test the Lid:** If you have any doubts about a seal, remove the screw band from the jar and gently lift the jar by the lid. A properly sealed jar should remain sealed, with the lid securely in place.

4. **Reprocessing Unsealed Jars:** If you find any unsealed jars, you have a few options. You can reprocess the contents in a new, sterilized jar with a fresh lid, following the original recipe and processing times. Alternatively, you can refrigerate the contents and use them within a reasonable time.

5. **Label and Store:** Once you've confirmed that your jars have proper seals, label them with the contents and date of canning. Store the jars in a cool, dark, and dry location, such as a pantry or cellar.

5.2. Dealing with Common Problems

Despite your best efforts, issues can occasionally arise in water bath canning. Here are some common problems and how to address them:

Problem: Jar Lids Don't Seal Properly

- **Solution:** If you have jars with unsealed lids, there are a few steps to take. First, allow the jars to cool completely. Then, check for the following issues:

- Ensure the jar rim was clean and free from food residue before applying the lid.

- Check that the screw band was fingertip tight, not overtightened, during the canning process.

- Make sure the flat metal lid was pre-warmed before application.

- Examine the rim of the jar for any nicks or irregularities that may have prevented a proper seal.

If the lids didn't seal due to a minor issue, you can reprocess the contents in a new, sterilized jar with a fresh lid following the original recipe and processing times. If the issue was not a minor one, such as significant damage to the rim or if the contents have spoiled, discard the contents, sterilize the jar, and start the process over with new contents and lids.

Problem: Jar Contents Have Unusual Color or Odor

- **Solution:** If you notice unusual colors, odors, or any signs of spoilage in the canned contents when you open the jar, do not consume the food. Discard it immediately. These are indicators of spoilage or contamination, and consuming such food can be harmful.

Problem: Food Siphoning During Processing

- **Solution:** Siphoning occurs when liquid is drawn out of the jars during processing, leaving inadequate headspace. To prevent siphoning:

- Follow recommended headspace guidelines for your recipe.

- Allow jars to cool undisturbed after processing. Rapid cooling can cause siphoning.

- Be gentle when moving the jars after processing.

If siphoning occurs, ensure the jar seals properly. If it does, the food inside is safe to eat. However, it may affect the appearance and texture of the contents.

Problem: Mold on Jar Tops or Contents

- **Solution:** If you notice mold on the jar tops or inside the contents after opening the jar, discard the contents immediately. Mold indicates spoilage and can be harmful if consumed. Ensure your jars and equipment are thoroughly cleaned and sterilized before canning.

Problem: Loss of Liquid During Storage

- **Solution:** Over time, some loss of liquid from canned goods may occur due to evaporation, which can lead to changes in texture or flavor. Ensure that you've followed recommended headspace guidelines and have used high-quality lids and bands. If you notice significant loss of liquid, it's best to consume or use the contents promptly.

In water bath canning, ensuring a proper seal and addressing common problems is essential for food safety and quality. Regularly inspect your canned goods, follow best practices, and don't hesitate to discard any items that show signs of spoilage or issues to protect your health and enjoyment of your preserved foods.

5.3. Best Practices for Long-Term Storage

Long-term storage is a key aspect of water bath canning, as it allows you to enjoy your preserved foods well into the future. Here are some best practices for long-term storage of your canned goods:

1. **Labeling and Organization:** Proper labeling is crucial for long-term storage. Clearly label each jar with the contents and the date of canning. Use a permanent marker or labels that won't smudge or fade over time. Organize your canned goods in a way that makes it easy to access

the oldest items first (a "first in, first out" system).

2. **Cool, Dark, and Dry:** Store your canned goods in a cool, dark, and dry location. A temperature between 50°F (10°C) and 70°F (21°C) is ideal. Avoid areas with temperature fluctuations or exposure to direct sunlight, as these can affect the quality of the contents.

3. **Shelf Stability:** Ensure that the shelves or storage area where you place your canned goods are stable and secure. Jars can be heavy, and a well-organized storage space minimizes the risk of accidents.

4. **Rotation:** Periodically rotate your stock of canned goods to use the oldest items first. This practice helps prevent waste and

ensures that you consume items while they are still at their best quality.

5. **Regular Inspection:** While your canned goods are in storage, inspect them periodically for any signs of spoilage or issues. This includes checking for unsealed lids, mold growth, unusual odors, or any visible damage to the jars.

6. **Storage Duration:** While most home-canned goods can be stored for 1-1.5 years or longer, it's a good practice to consume them within a reasonable time frame to enjoy the best flavor and quality. Keep an inventory of your canned goods and their estimated shelf life.

7. **Rotate High-Acid Foods:** High-acid foods like fruits, tomatoes,

and pickles generally have a shorter shelf life than low-acid foods. Rotate and consume these items more frequently to enjoy them at their peak quality.

8. **Use Proper Containers:** Consider using open shelving, wire racks, or sturdy wooden shelves for storage. These allow for proper air circulation and help prevent condensation, which can lead to rust and spoilage.

9. **Avoid Dampness:** Ensure that the storage area is free from dampness or high humidity. High moisture levels can lead to rust on lids and bands and promote mold growth on the jars.

10. **Re-check Seals:** Before using the contents of a jar, re-check the

seal to ensure it is intact. If a seal is compromised or the contents look or smell unusual, discard the food.

11. **Emergency Preparedness:** Having a well-stocked pantry of home-canned goods can be valuable for emergency preparedness. Make sure your storage area is accessible and well-organized for easy access during emergencies.

Following these best practices, you can confidently store your canned goods for an extended period while maintaining their safety and quality. Proper long-term storage ensures that your preserved foods are ready to enhance your meals and provide sustenance whenever you need them.

CHAPTER 6

Recipes for Water Bath Canning

6.1. Fruit Preserves

Strawberry Jam

Ingredients:

- 4 cups of ripe strawberries, hulled and crushed

- 4 cups of granulated sugar

- 1/4 cup of lemon juice

- 1 package (1.75 oz) of fruit pectin

Instructions:

1. Sterilize your canning jars, lids, and bands by boiling them in hot water or running them through the dishwasher with a sanitize cycle.

2. In a large, heavy-bottomed pot, combine the crushed strawberries and lemon juice. Stir in the fruit pectin.

3. Bring the strawberry mixture to a boil over medium-high heat, stirring frequently.

4. Once boiling, add the granulated sugar all at once, stirring constantly. Continue stirring until the mixture returns to a rolling boil.

5. Boil for 1-2 minutes or until the jam reaches your desired consistency. Stir frequently to prevent sticking.

6. Remove the pot from the heat
    and skim off any foam from the
    top of the jam.

7. Carefully ladle the hot jam into
    the prepared, hot canning jars,
    leaving the recommended
    headspace (typically 1/4 inch).
    Wipe the jar rims with a clean,
    damp cloth.

8. Place the flat metal lids on the
    jars, followed by screw bands,
    and tighten them fingertip-tight.

9. Process the jars in a water bath
    canner for 10-15 minutes,
    depending on your altitude. Start
    the timer once the water reaches
    a rolling boil.

10. Carefully remove the jars from
    the canner and place them on a
    clean towel or cooling rack.

11. Allow the jars to cool, undisturbed, for 12-24 hours. Check for proper seals, label the jars, and store in a cool, dark place.

6.2. Pickles and Relishes

Classic Dill Pickles

Ingredients:

- 3 lbs of small pickling cucumbers

- 6 cups of water

- 2 cups of white vinegar (5% acidity)

- 1/4 cup of pickling salt

- 4-6 cloves of garlic

- Fresh dill sprigs

- Red pepper flakes (optional for added heat)

Instructions:

1. Sterilize your canning jars, lids, and bands by boiling them in hot water or running them through the dishwasher with a sanitize cycle.

2. Wash the cucumbers thoroughly and trim the ends. Slice them into spears or leave them whole, as desired.

3. In a large pot, combine the water, vinegar, and pickling salt. Bring the mixture to a boil.

4. Place 1-2 garlic cloves, a sprig of fresh dill, and a pinch of red pepper flakes (if desired) in each sterilized jar.

5. Pack the cucumber spears or whole cucumbers into the jars, leaving about 1/2 inch of headspace.

6. Carefully ladle the hot vinegar mixture into each jar, ensuring that the cucumbers are fully covered, while maintaining the recommended headspace.

7. Wipe the jar rims with a clean, damp cloth.

8. Place the flat metal lids on the jars, followed by screw bands, and tighten them fingertip-tight.

9. Process the jars in a water bath canner for 10-15 minutes, depending on your altitude. Start the timer once the water reaches a rolling boil.

10. Carefully remove the jars from the canner and place them on a clean towel or cooling rack.

11. Allow the jars to cool, undisturbed, for 12-24 hours. Check for proper seals, label the jars, and store in a cool, dark place.

These recipes should help you get started with water bath canning and produce delicious fruit preserves and dill pickles. Adjust ingredients and seasonings to suit your taste preferences, and enjoy your homemade canned treats!

6.3. Jams and Jellies

Blueberry Jelly

Ingredients:

- 4 cups of blueberries

- 1/4 cup of lemon juice

- 1 package (1.75 oz) of fruit pectin

- 5 cups of granulated sugar

Instructions:

1. Sterilize your canning jars, lids, and bands by boiling them in hot water or running them through the dishwasher with a sanitize cycle.

2. In a large, heavy-bottomed pot, combine the blueberries and lemon juice. Crush the berries with a potato masher or fork to release their juice.

3. Stir in the fruit pectin and bring the mixture to a boil over medium-high heat, stirring frequently.

4. Once boiling, add the granulated
    sugar all at once, stirring
    constantly. Continue stirring
    until the mixture returns to a
    rolling boil.

5. Boil for 1-2 minutes or until the
    jelly reaches your desired
    consistency. Stir frequently to
    prevent sticking.

6. Remove the pot from the heat
    and skim off any foam from the
    top of the jelly.

7. Carefully ladle the hot jelly into
    the prepared, hot canning jars,
    leaving the recommended
    headspace (typically 1/4 inch).
    Wipe the jar rims with a clean,
    damp cloth.

8. Place the flat metal lids on the
    jars, followed by screw bands,
    and tighten them fingertip-tight.

9. Process the jars in a water bath canner for 10-15 minutes, depending on your altitude. Start the timer once the water reaches a rolling boil.

10. Carefully remove the jars from the canner and place them on a clean towel or cooling rack.

11. Allow the jars to cool, undisturbed, for 12-24 hours. Check for proper seals, label the jars, and store in a cool, dark place.

6.4. Salsas and Chutneys

Tomato Salsa

Ingredients:

- 10 cups of peeled, cored, and chopped tomatoes

- 5 cups of chopped onions

- 2.5 cups of chopped bell peppers

- 5 cups of cider vinegar (5% acidity)

- 2.5 cups of granulated sugar

- 2 tablespoons of pickling salt

- 4 cloves of garlic, minced

- 1 tablespoon of cumin

- 1 tablespoon of chili powder

- 1 teaspoon of red pepper flakes (adjust to taste)

Instructions:

1. Sterilize your canning jars, lids, and bands by boiling them in hot water or running them through the dishwasher with a sanitize cycle.

2. In a large pot, combine all the
    ingredients and bring the mixture
    to a boil.

3. Reduce the heat and simmer for
    10 minutes, stirring occasionally.

4. Carefully ladle the hot salsa into
    the prepared, hot canning jars,
    leaving the recommended
    headspace (typically 1/2 inch).
    Wipe the jar rims with a clean,
    damp cloth.

5. Place the flat metal lids on the
    jars, followed by screw bands,
    and tighten them fingertip-tight.

6. Process the jars in a water bath
    canner for 15-20 minutes,
    depending on your altitude. Start
    the timer once the water reaches
    a rolling boil.

7. Carefully remove the jars from
    the canner and place them on a
    clean towel or cooling rack.

8. Allow the jars to cool,
    undisturbed, for 12-24 hours.
    Check for proper seals, label the
    jars, and store in a cool, dark
    place.

These recipes for jams, jellies, salsas,
and chutneys can be customized to your
taste by adjusting spices and
ingredients. Proper canning and storage
will ensure you have delicious,
homemade condiments and spreads to
enjoy for months or even years to
come.

6.5. Tomato Sauce

Ingredients:

- 20 lbs of ripe tomatoes

- 2 cups of chopped onions

- 1 cup of chopped bell peppers

- 1 cup of chopped celery

- 4 cloves of garlic, minced

- 2 tablespoons of olive oil

- 2 tablespoons of granulated sugar (optional)

- 2 tablespoons of salt (adjust to taste)

- 2 teaspoons of dried basil

- 2 teaspoons of dried oregano

- 1/2 teaspoon of black pepper

- Lemon juice or citric acid for acidification

Instructions:

1. Sterilize your canning jars, lids, and bands by boiling them in hot

water or running them through the dishwasher with a sanitize cycle.

2. Prepare the tomatoes by blanching them in boiling water for 30 seconds, then immediately transferring them to an ice water bath to stop the cooking. This will make it easier to peel the tomatoes. Once peeled, chop the tomatoes.

3. In a large pot, heat the olive oil over medium heat. Add the chopped onions, bell peppers, and celery. Sauté for about 5-7 minutes until they become soft and translucent.

4. Add the minced garlic and continue to cook for another minute.

5. Add the chopped tomatoes to the pot, along with the sugar (if

using), salt, dried basil, dried oregano, and black pepper. Stir well.

6. Simmer the tomato mixture for about 30-45 minutes, or until it thickens to your desired consistency. Stir occasionally.

7. While the sauce is simmering, prepare your canning equipment, including the water bath canner, jars, lids, and bands.

8. Once the tomato sauce is ready, taste it and adjust the seasoning if necessary. If you prefer a more acidic sauce, add lemon juice or citric acid to each jar following the manufacturer's instructions for acidification. This is important for safe water bath canning.

9. Carefully ladle the hot tomato sauce into the prepared, hot

canning jars, leaving the recommended headspace (typically 1/2 inch). Wipe the jar rims with a clean, damp cloth.

10. Place the flat metal lids on the jars, followed by screw bands, and tighten them fingertip-tight.

11. Process the jars in a water bath canner for 35-45 minutes, depending on your altitude. Start the timer once the water reaches a rolling boil.

12. Carefully remove the jars from the canner and place them on a clean towel or cooling rack.

13. Allow the jars to cool, undisturbed, for 12-24 hours. Check for proper seals, label the jars, and store in a cool, dark place.

This tomato sauce is versatile and can be used in a variety of recipes. Canning tomato sauce allows you to enjoy the delicious flavor of garden-fresh tomatoes year-round.

CHAPTER 7

Beyond Water Bath Canning

7.1. Introduction to Pressure Canning

Pressure canning is a method of home food preservation that uses a specialized pressure canner to process low-acid foods, such as vegetables, meats, poultry, and seafood. It's a crucial technique for safely preserving foods that aren't suitable for water bath canning due to their low acidity. Pressure canning relies on higher temperatures and increased pressure to destroy harmful microorganisms like Clostridium botulinum spores, which can survive in low-acid environments.

Here are the basic steps and principles of pressure canning:

1. **Preparation:** Just like with water bath canning, start by gathering your equipment and preparing your canning jars, lids, and bands. Ensure your pressure canner is in good working order and has a functioning pressure gauge.

2. **Food Preparation:** Prepare the low-acid foods you intend to can. This may involve washing, cutting, blanching, or cooking the foods as required by the recipe.

3. **Jarring:** Fill hot, sterilized canning jars with the prepared food, leaving the recommended headspace specified in the recipe.

4. **Lid Placement:** Place sterilized
    flat metal lids on the jars and
    screw on sterilized screw bands
    just until they're fingertip-tight.

5. **Pressure Canner Loading:** Add
    water to your pressure canner as
    instructed by the manufacturer.
    Place the filled jars on the
    canner's rack or a trivet to ensure
    they don't touch the bottom of
    the canner. Properly secure the
    canner's lid.

6. **Venting and Building
    Pressure:** Follow the
    manufacturer's instructions to
    vent the canner by allowing
    steam to escape for a specified
    period. Once venting is
    complete, the canner's pressure
    will start to rise.

7. **Processing:** Once the pressure
    reaches the desired level, start

the timer for the recommended processing time as indicated in your canning recipe. Maintain the pressure throughout the processing time.

8. **Cooling and Unloading:** After the processing time, turn off the heat and allow the pressure to decrease naturally. Do not force-cool the canner. Once the pressure reaches zero and it is safe to open, carefully remove the jars.

9. **Cooling and Sealing:** Allow the jars to cool undisturbed for 12-24 hours. Check for proper seals, label the jars, and store them in a cool, dark place.

Pressure canning provides a safe way to preserve low-acid foods, extending their shelf life while maintaining quality. It's essential to follow tested recipes and canning guidelines to ensure the safety of the canned products.

7.2. Pressure Canning vs. Water Bath Canning

Pressure canning and water bath canning are both methods of home food preservation, but they are used for different types of foods due to their varying acidity levels. Here's a comparison of pressure canning and water bath canning:

Water Bath Canning:

- Suitable for high-acid foods like fruits, fruit preserves, jams, jellies, pickles, and some tomatoes.

- Uses boiling water to create a high-temperature environment

(212°F or 100°C) that is effective at destroying spoilage organisms and enzymes in high-acid foods.

- Typically, a water bath canner is used, which is a large pot with a rack to hold the jars. The water bath canner is heated on a stovetop.

- Processing times are relatively short, usually ranging from 5 to 20 minutes.

- Ideal for preserving the flavor and texture of high-acid foods.

- Requires acidic ingredients like lemon juice or vinegar to ensure safety.

Pressure Canning:

- Essential for low-acid foods like vegetables, meats, poultry, seafood, and some tomato products.

- Uses a pressure canner to create a higher-temperature, pressurized environment (typically 240-250°F or 116-121°C) to safely destroy harmful microorganisms, including Clostridium botulinum spores, which are not effectively destroyed in a water bath canner.

- The pressure canner is a specialized piece of equipment designed for safe high-pressure canning. It has a pressure gauge and safety features.

- Processing times are longer, often ranging from 20 minutes to several hours, depending on the food and jar size.

- Preserves low-acid foods with longer shelf life and can be used for creating soups, stews, and other ready-to-eat meals.

- Does not require additional acidification because of the high-temperature processing.

The choice between pressure canning and water bath canning depends on the type of food you want to preserve. High-acid foods are suitable for water bath canning, while low-acid foods require pressure canning to ensure safety and quality. It's crucial to follow trusted recipes and canning guidelines for each method to prevent foodborne illnesses and spoilage.

7.3. Foods Suitable for Pressure Canning

Pressure canning is the ideal method for safely preserving low-acid foods, as it uses high temperatures and pressure to destroy harmful microorganisms, such as Clostridium botulinum spores, which can thrive in low-acid environments. Here is a list of foods that are suitable for pressure canning:

1. **Vegetables:** Pressure canning is commonly used for vegetables, both single vegetables and mixed vegetable combinations. Examples include green beans, carrots, peas, corn, potatoes, and mixed vegetable medleys.

2. **Meats:** Pressure canning is excellent for preserving meats, including poultry (chicken, turkey), red meats (beef, pork, lamb), and game meats (venison, elk). Meats are often canned in chunks, strips, or ground form.

3. **Poultry:** Chicken and turkey can be pressure canned in various forms, including whole pieces,

chunks, and ground. Canned poultry can be used in soups, stews, and casseroles.

4. **Seafood:** Pressure canning is suitable for canning various types of seafood, such as salmon, tuna, mackerel, and shellfish. Canned seafood is often used in salads, sandwiches, and seafood chowders.

5. **Soups and Stews:** You can create and can your own soups and stews with a combination of vegetables, meats, and seasonings. Canning soups and stews is convenient for quick and hearty meals.

6. **Chili:** Chili can be pressure canned and enjoyed as a ready-to-serve meal. You can customize the ingredients and spice level to suit your taste.

7. **Spaghetti Sauce:** Homemade spaghetti sauce with meat or vegetables can be pressure canned for quick pasta dinners.

8. **Beans:** Various types of beans, such as black beans, kidney beans, and pinto beans, can be pressure canned for convenience and versatility in cooking.

9. **Grains:** Some grains, like barley or rice, can be canned alongside other ingredients in soups and stews.

10. **Broths and Stocks:** Chicken, beef, or vegetable broths and stocks can be pressure canned for use as a base in various recipes.

11. **Tomato Products:** Low-acid tomato products like tomato sauce, crushed tomatoes, or

diced tomatoes can be safely
pressure canned.

12. **Sauces:** Beyond tomato-based
    sauces, you can pressure can a
    variety of other sauces, such as
    barbecue sauce and hot sauce.

13. **Baby Food:** Homemade baby
    food can be pressure canned for
    a convenient and nutritious
    option for infants.

14. **Fruits (Non-Acidic):** While
    fruits are generally water bath
    canned, there are some
    exceptions, like figs and Asian
    pears, which are low in acidity
    and require pressure canning.

It's important to follow tested and
trusted pressure canning recipes and
guidelines to ensure the safety and
quality of canned low-acid foods.
Additionally, be sure to use a properly
functioning pressure canner and

maintain the correct pressure and processing times as specified in your chosen recipes. Properly canned low-acid foods have a longer shelf life and can be used in a variety of recipes to make meal preparation more convenient.

CHAPTER 8

Storing and Using Canned Goods

8.1. Labeling and Storage Tips

Proper labeling and storage are essential for maintaining the quality and safety of your home-canned goods. Here are some tips for labeling and storing your canned foods:

Labeling Tips:

1. **Label Contents and Date:** Clearly label each jar with the contents and the date it was canned. This helps you easily identify what's inside and track the age of your canned goods.

2. **Use Waterproof Ink:** Write your labels with a waterproof or permanent marker to ensure they don't smudge or fade over time.

3. **Include Any Variations:** If you've made different variations of a particular food, such as different spice levels for salsa, specify the variation on the label.

4. **Include Processing Information:** Note the processing method used (water bath canning or pressure canning) if it's not obvious from the recipe. This information can be important if you're trying to decide how to use the contents.

Storage Tips:

1. **Cool, Dark, and Dry:** Store your canned goods in a cool, dark, and dry location, such as a pantry or cellar. Avoid areas

with temperature fluctuations, direct sunlight, or high humidity.

2. **Shelf Stability:** Ensure that the shelves or storage area where you place your canned goods are stable and secure. Jars can be heavy, and a well-organized storage space minimizes the risk of accidents.

3. **Rotation:** Periodically rotate your stock of canned goods to use the oldest items first. This practice helps prevent waste and ensures that you consume items while they are still at their best quality.

4. **Regular Inspection:** While your canned goods are in storage, inspect them periodically for any signs of spoilage or issues. This includes checking for unsealed lids, mold growth, unusual

odors, or any visible damage to the jars.

5. **Storage Duration:** While most home-canned goods can be stored for 1-1.5 years or longer, it's a good practice to consume them within a reasonable time frame to enjoy the best flavor and quality. Keep an inventory of your canned goods and their estimated shelf life.

6. **Rotate High-Acid Foods:** High-acid foods like fruits, tomatoes, and pickles generally have a shorter shelf life than low-acid foods. Rotate and consume these items more frequently to enjoy them at their peak quality.

7. **Use Proper Containers:** Consider using open shelving, wire racks, or sturdy wooden shelves for storage. These allow

for proper air circulation and help prevent condensation, which can lead to rust and spoilage.

8. **Avoid Dampness:** Ensure that the storage area is free from dampness or high humidity. High moisture levels can lead to rust on lids and bands and promote mold growth on the jars.

9. **Re-check Seals:** Before using the contents of a jar, re-check the seal to ensure it is intact. If a seal is compromised or the contents look or smell unusual, discard the food.

Following these labeling and storage tips, you can maintain the safety and quality of your home-preserved foods and enjoy them for an extended period.

8.2. Creative Ways to Use Home-Preserved Foods

Home-canned goods offer a world of culinary possibilities. Here are some creative ways to use your home-preserved foods:

1. **Salsas and Relishes:** Use homemade salsas and relishes as flavorful toppings for grilled meats, fish, and vegetables. They also work well as condiments for tacos, sandwiches, and hot dogs.

2. **Fruit Preserves:** Beyond spreading fruit preserves on toast or biscuits, incorporate them into your cooking. For example, mix fruit preserves into marinades for grilled chicken or glazes for roasted meats.

3. **Tomato Sauce:** Homemade tomato sauce is a versatile

ingredient for making pasta dishes, lasagna, and pizza. It can also serve as a base for chili and various soups.

4. **Pickles:** Pickles add a delightful crunch and tang to sandwiches, burgers, and salads. You can also chop pickles finely and use them in potato salad or coleslaw.

5. **Jams and Jellies:** Jams and jellies are not just for breakfast. They can be used as glazes for baked goods, sweeteners for marinades, or additions to cheese platters.

6. **Canned Vegetables:** Incorporate canned vegetables like green beans, carrots, or peas into casseroles, stir-fries, and soups. They provide a convenient source of vegetables for recipes.

7. **Canned Meats:** Canned meats, such as chicken or beef, are perfect for making quick sandwiches, quesadillas, or savory pies. They can also be added to salads for a protein boost.

8. **Chutneys:** Chutneys can be used as condiments for roasted meats, curries, or grilled cheese sandwiches. They add a burst of flavor with their sweet and tangy profile.

9. **Tomato Products:** Canned tomatoes, like diced or crushed tomatoes, are excellent for making homemade tomato-based sauces, stews, and chili. They can also be used as a base for curry dishes.

10. **Canned Fruits:** Canned fruits can be used in desserts like

cobblers, crisps, and fruit tarts. They also make a convenient addition to smoothies and oatmeal.

11. **Canned Broths:** Homemade broths and stocks can enhance the flavor of soups, risottos, and sauces. They serve as a foundational ingredient for many recipes.

12. **Preserved Eggs:** If you've preserved eggs, they can be used in baking, quiches, and omelets.

13. **Chili:** Home-canned chili can be used as a topping for hot dogs or as a base for chili mac and other one-pot meals.

The key is to get creative and experiment with your home-preserved foods. They can add unique flavors and a personal touch to your culinary creations.